BREATH

BREATH

THE YOGIC PRIME

EXPLORATION, MEDITATIONS AND STORIES ON THE MAT

GABRIEL AZOULAY

iUniverse, Inc.
New York Lincoln Shanghai

Breath
The Yogic Prime

Copyright © 2007 by Gabriel Azoulay

iUniverse books may be ordered through booksellers or by contacting:

iUniverse
2021 Pine Lake Road, Suite 100
Lincoln, NE 68512
www.iuniverse.com
1-800-Authors (1-800-288-4677)

ISBN-13: 978-0-595-42595-2 (pbk)
ISBN-13: 978-0-595-86923-7 (ebk)
ISBN-10: 0-595-42595-X (pbk)
ISBN-10: 0-595-86923-8 (ebk)

Printed in the United States of America

I would like to thank each of the students, those who happened to be in my classes before, those who take my classes or seminars now, and those who I will meet in the future. You are my best teachers.

I also would like to thank my parents and grandparents, who taught me to seek more than the obvious.

There are key people who read my early chapters and who pushed me to continue despite any hesitation on my part. Without your support, this book may have stayed an idea.

I would like to thank each of the students, those who happened to be in my classes before, those who take my classes or seminars now, and those who I will meet in the future. You are my best teachers.

I also would like to thank my parents and grandparents, who taught me to seek more than the obvious.

There are key people who read my early chapters and who pushed me to continue despite any hesitation on my part. Without your support, this book may have stayed an idea.

CONTENTS

INTRODUCTION

After following the tale of a king who lived for one thousand years, I entered my college library and sought out as many books as I could on India's culture and history. I was astounded to find rich, ancient philosophical answers to questions that had been circulating in my head from early childhood. These answers, I was to discover over years of teaching and practicing, have a thread behind them, a unifying theme. This thread is our breath. While memorizing long verses, ancient yogis learned to control their breath, and in that practice something magical happened. Breath was recognized as the liberator of the true body and inner being.

Breath can neither be seen, nor touched, yet it can be felt and manipulated. Breath keeps the body active and alive as well as connects us to those around us. Modern yoga focuses on breath and body postures. While the mind is able to observe the transformations that are possible via the body, the breath connects mind and body. Breath grounds us in the moment, without judging ourselves, or another. It is this practice of non-judging that evokes 'samadhi' the Sanskrit term for enlightenment, or in a more direct translation 'neutral vision.' (sama = same/neautral dhi = to see).

The stories, anecdotes, and personal experiences in this volume touch on the mystery of breath. Imagine you are taking a yoga class; follow the book with the softness and open mind that you allow while listening and breathing in class. Each chapter is a meditation on its own—with a story, exploration, or new philosophical perspective. You can pick up the book, read any chapter, and see how you react to it throughout the day. Some stories may come to mind again in moments of tension or joy. They may offer a new perspective or a different outlook at the events you are facing.

I learned these stories through many years of thought and exploration. They have changed my practice and deepened my appreciation of the unique and wonderful gift of yoga.

I honor the place in you of light, love, peace, and joy.

I honor this place in you, and when you are in that place and I am in that place,

There is only one of us. (loose translation of the word *Namaste*)

INTRODUCTION

After following the tale of a king who lived for one thousand years, I entered my college library and sought out as many books as I could on India's culture and history. I was astounded to find rich, ancient philosophical answers to questions that had been circulating in my head from early childhood. These answers, I was to discover over years of teaching and practicing, have a thread behind them, a unifying theme. This thread is our breath. While memorizing long verses, ancient yogis learned to control their breath, and in that practice something magical happened. Breath was recognized as the liberator of the true body and inner being.

Breath can neither be seen, nor touched, yet it can be felt and manipulated. Breath keeps the body active and alive as well as connects us to those around us. Modern yoga focuses on breath and body postures. While the mind is able to observe the transformations that are possible via the body, the breath connects mind and body. Breath grounds us in the moment, without judging ourselves, or another. It is this practice of non-judging that evokes 'samadhi' the Sanskrit term for enlightenment, or in a more direct translation 'neutral vision.' (sama = same/neautral dhi = to see).

The stories, anecdotes, and personal experiences in this volume touch on the mystery of breath. Imagine you are taking a yoga class; follow the book with the softness and open mind that you allow while listening and breathing in class. Each chapter is a meditation on its own—with a story, exploration, or new philosophical perspective. You can pick up the book, read any chapter, and see how you react to it throughout the day. Some stories may come to mind again in moments of tension or joy. They may offer a new perspective or a different outlook at the events you are facing.

I learned these stories through many years of thought and exploration. They have changed my practice and deepened my appreciation of the unique and wonderful gift of yoga.

I honor the place in you of light, love, peace, and joy.

I honor this place in you, and when you are in that place and I am in that place,

There is only one of us. (loose translation of the word *Namaste)*

I. ONE BREATH

"A beginning yoga student walks up to the teacher after his first class, and says 'Yoga is hard. My body is so stiff and my thoughts are everywhere.'"

My class challenged my students, and I share one of my favorite stories.

"The yoga teacher smiles and says 'Don't worry, that will pass.'

"A few months later the same student comes up to the teacher and says: 'Yoga is so wonderful! My body feels so light, there are times I feel I could walk over water. My mind is so focused; there are moments I feel I am centered in heaven with the angels.'

"The yoga teacher smiles, and says 'Don't worry, that will pass.'"

Kathy, one of my students, lies on her back in *savasana* [corpse pose], having moved into a centered peace—a physical release and surrender—due in part to the yoga class and in part to the calm setting of her retreat, which is away from the clatter of her everyday existence.

"You made me see my father," she says with a smile as her eyes sparkle like the early evening stars.

"I did?" I ask as I walk over to her and return her smile.

"In your story about the student," she continues while looking me straight in the eyes, "when you said he feels like he is among the angels, I could see my father."

Kathy's eyes begin to well up.

"I'm sorry," she confesses. "I can't stop crying."

As tears moisten her cheeks, her face smiles and her voice softens. She stands with her shoulders relaxed, spine straight, and neck visible and true.

As Kathy engages her body and emotions, she is surprised at how selfless she actually feels. Talking about her father while taking full, calming breaths offers her the ability to relax as she takes in everything she feels.

"He passed away last year, and I came here this week to connect—not to move on, but to move with," she explains. "Seeing him today—and I have seen him in other ways throughout this past year—I know he is with me, and that story made me feel the energy of his love. I know he loved me in spite of any problems. I feel it now. Thank you so much. Thank you."

Chances are you have had a moment of such connection. It could have been in your yoga class, when your child was born, when you accomplished something that you worked really hard at, or when you fell in love. Often in this connection, we feel a sense of identity dissolution as we surrender to the moment, open up to love, and realize the divine. This connection draws us into partnership, parenthood, and the ability to share love with the world.

The art of yoga reveals this connection through its teaching on breath. At first, breath connects the actions of the mind with the interactions of the body, and from there, we can relax into this very moment quicker and easier. When we find ourselves grounded in the present a transforming gift is presented. We unravel all our potential.

When centered on the breath, you can face habitual thought patterns, be inspired to new views of reality, and change behavior patterns. You can, learn to extend the capacity of your breath, such as resting under water for long periods of time, however, these feats are difficult to accomplish. If your body does not receive a fresh supply of oxygen in as little as five minutes, you will die. While breath is more vital than food or water, we spend very little time reflecting on, or practicing to know our breath.

Yoga philosophy describes three states of knowledge: waking, dreaming, and deep sleep. Each of these states has a corresponding physical attribute through which we come to understand the world around us. The first state, waking, has the physical body as its corresponding attribute. In the second state, dreaming, the corresponding attribute is the subtle body, where thoughts, emotions, desire, and other internal imagery (such as day dreams, visions, etc.) are experienced and manifested. The third state, deep sleep, is referred to as the causal body and is where you experience your true self, beyond mind and body, beyond name and address. This state, which can occur during meditation, ecstatic dance, or spontaneously, is also referred to as 'enlightment' or 'samadhi.'

You can practice for the rest of your life and never achieve this so-called 'samadhi.' You can achieve this recognition (as others have) in a few hours time. Yoga, on the other hand, is when we recognize all three states with each passing moment *and* engage in the drama around us.

Yoga philosophy cares little about the accomplishments we can enact with our bodies, the achievements we can master with our minds. And yet we have a body, and through this body we can experience so much. We have a mind, which can discover even the smallest of atoms. What we choose to focus on, we achieve. Yet Yoga chooses to guide us past the temporary existence of our body/mind, while we discover our full capacities. Your breath is the quickest compass to this recognition. Whether you choose to win a race, or write a novel, connecting with the breath prepares the body and centers the mind. While you continue in your activities, your breath reflects the connection around you.

There are times when you walk into your house after a stressful, busy day, your thoughts are engaged in the day's events, and your physical body is tired and tense. As you settle in for the evening, the energy in your house only accentuates the tension you feel, and your partner or kids easily anger you.

Yet no matter how arduous your day has been, you can be aware of your breath and walk into your house centered. You are already breathing, and so when you are conscious of breath—by inhaling and exhaling deep into your belly—your gross body softens and your subtle body centers in the now. The day's events and other thoughts can still remain, yet you will stay grounded through your breathing, which occurs in the moment. From such a center, you will respond to the energy in your house in a completely different way. Your centeredness of mind and body, the gross and the subtle, will center your home.

This diaphragmatic breathing is the natural pattern of our breath. Yet as you grow older, you get caught up in your anxieties (for example, what you need from others, what others think of your behavior, where you want to go in the future, what has happened in the past, are you successful, or are you loved enough). Your breath becomes constricted and short, and these gross body changes are magnified by subtle body fears.

It is your life. In this body, with this mind, you only have one life to live. Your life passes by—breath by breath, moment by moment. By inhaling and exhaling, you hold both the life and the death of your mind and your body body, opening as the infinite spirit that lives all. Can you live your life fully, recognizing the causal, yet with each breath, offering everything you can through your gross and subtle, as if it were your last breath? Will you experience life in its fullness, or will you prefer to dull your senses by watching TV, drinking beer, sleeping hurriedly, rising to work, and then repeating the cycle the next day? Follow your breath, and it will guide you to happiness. Follow your thoughts, and you will stay in the cycle.

Step out of the circle of fear, and pay attention to your breath. Let it spiral down into your belly as you inhale. Let it rise back as you exhale. Continue your activities breathing this way. There is a different quality in the way you sit, stand or walk, a more focused view, perspective or idea. For fifteen minutes a day, breathe full and deep and note in a journal your gross physical changes, your subtle emotions or thoughts, and any experiences you may have had in recognizing the causal, the expression of non-separation around you.

2. CONNECT

It has been a long day. The phone never stopped ringing. The emails kept coming. Clients were not satisfied. A sales deal you have been working on for a month fell through. Construction caused a traffic jam. Your children discovered the Swiss chocolate you save for special occasions, consequentially sending them on a sugar high for most of the afternoon.

As you sit in your car, you ponder if you truly want to go to class.

You inhale.

As the air circles in your *gross*, or physical, body, a sense of lightness begins to fill your *subtle*, or inner, body. Oxygen settles in your belly. Assisted by your intercostals muscles, air fills the diaphragm, chest, and shoulders. A rush of positive calm descends upon your nervous system.

You exhale.

You might not be able to control the world, but you can control the way you breathe in this world, and often, that will change *your* world. You make it to class.

"Diaphragmatic breathing has far-reaching benefits, which are both physical and emotional," explains the yoga instructor to his class.

His baritone voice rings like ancient Buddhist gongs and vibrates in the ears of his resting students.

"Belly breathing reduces the cortisol level in our blood," he continues. "Cortisol is the adrenaline hormone associated with obesity, memory loss, and depression. As you breathe into your lower torso, your heart rate and blood pressure find their natural balance as they restore a sense of peace in your minds."

"Watching my baby sister breathe helped me to learn the value of yoga breathing," he observes didactically. "On her back, completely present or maybe completely oblivious, she was breathing into her belly. As you lie on your back, let your shoulders relax into the floor, and place a palm on your belly. Imagine your belly is a balloon, and as you inhale, fill it with air. As you exhale, let the belly relax. Imagine the soft breathing of an infant. Let the oxygen fill your belly, which should be round as a balloon, and allow the act of exhalation to relax your body deeper. With a conscious awareness of our breath, we can elicit the physical sensation of peace, even in the midst of an emotional or physical storm."

With each syllable muscles unwind, with each word a new bodies settle more.

"Breathing into the belly activates the diaphragmatic muscle, massages the digestive organs, and releases tension from the intercostal muscles, increasing breath capacity. Deeper breathing stimulates movement in the lower back, fostering an overall sense of calmness. While it may take a few days, weeks, or even months before you are able to release your preconceived notions about relaxing the belly and your habitual patterns of constricting your abdominal muscles and enjoy a deep, full breath, right now your breath is full, your body relaxed, and your mind at ease."

8

Use this as a breathing exercise: Pull a cushion from your couch and allow your entire spine to rest on the cushion. If you need support for your head, a blanket is very handy. This should be very comfortable, so create any adjustments you need if you are not comfortable. Your legs can stretch straight out in front. They can bend at the knees, cross at the shins, or be placed in *supta baddha konasana* (the outside of the feet touching, knees butterfly to the floor). You might notice the upward tilt of your pelvic bone, something that is very similar to the tilt we naturally create in order to sit up straight. This tilt releases the lower spine, and in return, releases tension from your lower belly muscles.

Close your eyes, and begin to relax into the pillow. Feel the support and the safety under your body. Focus on your breath. When do you inhale? When do you exhale? Even though this focus may create a desire to control, free yourself from the natural urge to manipulate or control your breath. Do not judge the way your body is breathing. It might be erratic or strained in the beginning. These are all natural movements of your breath. Honor them, relax into them, and just pay attention. When is breath moving into your body? When is breath leaving your body?

As you breathe, relax your jaw, close your mouth, smile, place your tongue on the roof of your palate, and let your breath move in and out of your nose. As you relax into your breathing, it moves deep into your belly. Feel your belly muscles. What are they doing when the body inhales? How do they relax when you exhale? Feel your belly, and appreciate your body's natural ability to relax.

Inhale, and allow your belly to expand. Let your breath fill your lungs and the back of your shoulders. Exhale, and allow your belly muscles to push more air out of the body. Inhale, and repeat the process for fifteen minutes, breathing deeply and fully.

This process will help you become more familiar with the muscular movements of your belly as it interacts with your breath. As you master the ability to relax into this natural movement of your body, you'll be able to access the same awareness when you are walking, talking, driving, sitting, running, or practicing your yoga. Feel the breath moving down the body, filling the belly, and moving up the spine as the belly dissolves. Try breathing this way throughout your day.

Breathing in. Breathing out. Moment by moment. Breath by breath.

3. WHY FIGHT?

Blake has been holding his *virabhadrasana* (warrior pose) for two minutes now, but for him, it seems like eternity. His right quadriceps muscle burns. His breath wavers between smooth and erratic. His mind directs profanities at the instructor, and his spirit threatens to abandon him. Despite this internal chaos, Blake is determined.

"I'm going to stick it through," he tells himself above the flowing river of violent internal remarks.

"Rise above the battleground," the teacher's voice rings through his churning thoughts. "You have already won all of your battles. Relax into the moment. Breathe through the tension. It is your mind that doubts that your body is ready to transform."

"Yeah, right!" Blake's brain shoots back.

"Inhale," the instructor commands and encourages. "Nice holding. Exhale. Release into *chaturanga dandasana* [low push-up pose]."

As Blake lowers his body into a push-up position, his body exhales into surrender. The floor seems very appealing from this vantage point. His mind is ready to lie down, let go, and surrender, but that would be giving up. There is no giving up in this body.

"Let your breath push your spine up into *urdhva mukha svanasana* [upward-facing dog pose]," the instructor continues. "Use your thighs to lift the heart."

The instructor is trying to paint a picture, but for Blake, in the throws of the battle, the image seems blurry. He allows his body to move while allowing the breath to find its own rhythm.

"Let your thighs take you back into adho mukha svanasana [downward-facing dog pose] as you exhale."

"I'll stay right here," Blake's mind opines, as Blake's body follows the directives. The battle still rages.

"Bring your left foot forward. Lift it, kick it, and step it as far forward as you can. Plant your right foot into the earth, and blossom with your arms into virabhadrasana 1."

"Oh, no," Blake's mind protests. "Not the left side."

Sweat pours down Blake's face, and his eyes tingle, but unbeknownst to him, his skin shines.

"In the great battle between the gods, Shiva received a terrible message," the instructor narrates as his students hold the pose. "His wife—his cohort and his dancing partner—had been killed in battle. Overwhelmed with grief and shocked with passing anger, Shiva tore a lock from his hair and threw it to the ground. When the lock hit the earth, it was transformed into two new deities, a warrior god and an avenging goddess. The warrior god is known as Virabhadra, and the goddess is Kali. All life is preceded by death. Rather than fearing it, accept the cycle of life and the humor in the face of challenge. Allow the warrior in you to battle against your ego. Desire to reject death and only hold onto life. Inhale the beauty of life, and exhale your fear of death as you release into chaturanga dandasana."

With his mind attuned to the story, Blake's body moves with his breath, and as he transitions into a low push-up, he is surprised to notice how light and calm his left side seems in comparison to the right.

"Come into *balasana* [child's pose]."

Children play whether in joy or when in anger. Let the child in you come forward. Faced with a physical challenge, you either move with forceful intention to fight your way through or you come out of the pose running away from the situation. Fight or flight syndrome perpetuates the cyclic tension in your life, the constant battle between one direction and another. You feel lost in your own needs and your own desires as if the cause of this tension emanates from outside yourself. You see you are so enclosed in your own realm that you don't realize that you are oblivious to a third choice—the choice to breathe and relax, to smile and be, to accept the moment just as it is while feeling your body, and to connect your self-identity with the whole universe.

4.   TO SIT IN AGONY OR MOVE ECSTATICALLY?

In our fast-paced, work-laden, success-driven, ego-centered modern world, individuals often look for a quick fix formula. They want something they can take, do, exchange, or contemplate on their way to the next meeting, practice, affair, or engagement.

For example, Martin, who is working full time at a fast-paced Internet sales company, is disappointed by his inability to maintain a regular gym routine. He has been reading about yoga for some time, and he has noticed the physical and emotional changes in colleagues who have begun yoga practice. He decides to go to a class. He finds one at his local gym and eagerly prepares himself mentally to show up.

The instructor, a full-bodied middle-aged woman, is seated in a cross-legged position that Martin realizes he will not be able to do. He tries very hard to overcome his self-consciousness as he looks around the room at the seemingly well-adapted students.

Recognizing her new student, the instructor smiles at Martin and says, "If you fold your blanket and sit on its edge, your body will experience more comfort."

Martin follows with the suggestion, and to his pleasant surprise, his body settles with considerable ease. Now, his pelvic floor can support his lower back as the vertebrae stack along their axis.

"Yoga postures, or *asana* in Sanskrit have been explored and developed by the ancient yoga masters as a physical support for seated meditation," explains the instructor. "The root for the word *asana* is the sound 'aa-s' which means 'to sit.'"

"I sit all day long in a comfortable leather chair," Martin thinks to himself. "Why work out to sit back down? I don't know how long I can keep this up without some extra support. I'm not so sure about these so-called ancient masters."

"Modern and ancient masters will sit for hours without moving, maintaining a straight spine," the instructor continues. "Average adults find it extremely difficult to sit for a few minutes without back support. While sitting with the spine relaxed, yet straight, breath can move deeply into the belly, filling the lungs and abdomen with ease. Remember that if you cannot breathe easily and deeply while in your posture, it is an indication that you are not in the most comfortable alignment. Let your breath lead, and let your body follow. All that matters is your breath. Let's come onto our palms and knees in a table position."

"I never thought about my breath like that before," Martin moves his body forward, with a curious look he follows the instructors movements.

I see the mind as a function of the ego. We would rather continue to immerse ourselves in our thoughts, reassuring ourselves of our immediate existence, than let go and simply watch the thoughts. Like a child learning to use his fingers, your mind uses imaginary fingers to reach out and grab the next thought, the next project, and the next idea. This incessant need to grasp is an indication of the ego's need for self-validation. Your thoughts move, changing form and content and continually flowing and dancing, but these thoughts exist only inside your personal realm unless expressed. Until then, the world is oblivious to them and they remained trapped, constantly recycling around inside your head. What might happen when you release your grasp on them and enjoy the silence?

Three yoga students decided to explore the realm of silent meditation. They agreed to be silent for a full week. On the first evening, they sat together reading by the light of a candle. A strong wind pierced through their window and blew out the candle.

"Oh, no," one of the students said. "The candle went out."

"We are not suppose to be speaking," replied the second.

"Wow," commented the third. "I am the only one who did not speak."

Modern culture tells you to fill every space with something. Often people tell you, "Don't just sit there. Get up and do something. Reach out and hold onto something. Touch yourself so you know you are still here. Speak and show others that you have not left." What would happen if you just sat there, instead of worrying about how others view you?

When you choose to be silent with the world, you begin to notice how distracting your conversations become. The philosophy of yoga believes that conversation is tension while silence is communication. Many spiritual teachers often challenge their students to step into the world of silence. For example, sit with your lover feel the connection beyond the superficial separation of two different bodies. Notice what happens when you interact with your friends without diluting the moment and without a barrage of plans, ideas, suggestions, and constant chit-chat. It is only then that you can let your natural light—your essence—shine through.

In the silence, you have an opportunity to discover a deeper interaction, rather than continue listening to the changing thoughts in your head. As you move out of the noise of your mind and into the silence, there can be some questions that pop into your mind:

"How can I define this experience?"

"Am I really present in this moment, or am I holding on to past ideas or future plans?"

"Am I truly present in the moment, or am I searching for a better connection?"

As these questions come, accept the fluctuating shift of your awareness; honor your need to be noticed, which validates your ego; embrace your faults and your strengths; and relax into this moment as it is. Don't change it. You can do that by focusing on your breathing. Relax into the silence by breathing this moment into your body. Breathe it fully, and deepen your awareness, *right now*.

To be, or not to be?

Be in silence, and you will not have to question.

5. PRACTICE

Morning light has barely pierced the pursed horizon's lips, revealing Mother Earth's spring colors. In celebration of the great Mother, I join a group of yogis and yoginis in the ancient dance of Sun Salutations. Uniting the flow of breath with the body, and bridging culture and spirit, man and woman, stranger and friend, the group gather to honor the ancient practice by moving through 108 Sun Salutations.

One hundred and eight because of the 108 *Upanishads*.

One hundred and eight because you are, a star. With your five senses, you are, a five pointed star. Take the pentagon, add the two adjacent angles, the total is 108.

One hundred and eight because when you multiply the number of the Sanskrit characters (fifty-four) by two in light of every element containing both *Shiva* (the divine masculine) and *Shakti* (the divine feminine), you get 108.

One hundred and eight because when you multiply the twelve houses in the sky, representing the horoscope, and the nine different planets, you get 108.

One hundred and eight because there are 108 beads in a *mala* [prayer beads]. Practice is shedding off your sense of separateness by connecting your mind and body with the larger force of the universe, called Prana. The above examples help to inspire us to move into our own practice.

In the early hours of this Saturday morning, the class moves through *suryanmaskar A;*sun salutations A, moving as individuals, yet centered on breath. There are various bodies of various shapes and backgrounds, but each person is connected to an energy; each individual is an expression of the divine; the group is all one, dissolved in love.

As you practice 108 Sun Salutations, your surroundings can easily distract you.

"I'm too weak," your mind complains to your body.

"What am I doing here?" your mind fights as you try to remain present in the moment.

"Wow, that person is moving so beautifully. Let me imitate them."

Stay focused on the breath, and the mind's chatter will fade.

"But this is 108 Sun Salutations," you say. "Who has time for breath awareness? Inhale? Exhale? Let me just finish."

Who will lead? The mind or the body?

Come back. The movements, like words on paper, do not change.

Come back. You just started.

Come back. Take a slow, deep breath, and let the breath, not your mind, move you.

As we have mentioned earlier, your mind travels through the past, the present, and the future. When it is guided and reined in through any practice, your mind experiences its witness quality, which is beyond mind and body. There is resistance, because your ego enjoys its self-assurance through the shifting thought paradigms. Like a child who constantly seeks attention, the ego finds many excuses to postpone practice.

By practicing being present and moving through your mental resistance, you face your worries and your anxieties, your insecurities and your fears, your needs and your dreams. Above all, it reveals the infinite possibilities that lie underneath the layer of thoughts, emotions and physical sensations. Yoga practice can also been seen as the uncovering of our individual capacity, discovering our strengths and persisting through our weaknesses. While we are all connected, we are each unique, special, indispensable, and irreplaceable. Our gifts and talents for the world are also unique and irreplaceable. Only you can uncover them, only you can find them out, as the best guru is in you.

6. WAKE UP

The *Upanishads* claim that our universe arose from the sound, *om. Om* is one sound in Sanskrit that has no seed. It is said that the ancient yogis sat and meditated, and in this connected state they heard and felt the vibrations that maintain our world.

Say *om* to yourself. Feel the vibrations in the belly as you begin with the "aw," then feel them move into the chest as you pronounce the "o," and finally feel them in the throat as you close with the "um."

The sound for knowledge is the word bood. *The word* Buddha *can thus be translated as someone who knows. To that extent we are all Buddhas. We are each someone with knowledge.*

The first Buddha, Siddhartha Gautama, was once asked if he was a god.

The Buddha smiled and said, "No."

"Are you a saint?" he was asked.

"No," said the Buddha with a smile.

"What are you?" he was asked.

"I am awake."

Are you awake? Are your physical, subtle, and causal bodies aware of each other? If you die tomorrow, would you be satisfied in knowing that you offered everything you could today? It's OK if the answer is no; you still have this moment—right now. Pick up the phone and call your lover, your mother, your brother, or your friend. Connect with your father, your sister, the person next to you, or a complete stranger. If you want to see your dreams materialize, now is as good a time as any. In fact, if not now, when?

There are many levels to being awake. Obviously, you are currently awake and reading. You are cognizant of the chair, floor, couch, or bed. You are aware of your music, your lover, the TV, or silence. Today, you worked or went to school, ate, and spoke with others. You drove, walked, ran, or pedaled from one place to another. You could argue this was all a dream;

in a dream we can be afraid, we can touch, we can taste, we can smell, so it could be a dream as well.

It could be.

But it is not.

Or maybe it is?

Let's agree that you are awake—awake to explore where you are and what your true gift to this world is. What is the true essence of your being? Are you feeling your body? Are you focusing on breath? Are you meditating on the infinite? Or maybe you are stuck in the constant cycle of your thoughts? Perhaps you are overwhelmed with your emotions and responsibilities?

You can get caught up in *samsara* [the world of illusion], a conditioned behavior that focuses on the monotony of life and the routine of your days. And even though you are awake, you move through life as if it were a dream. One day, you awaken from this stupor to realize that you are much older and the goals you really wanted to accomplish are much harder to begin.

Breath is both a bridge between the mind-body connection and an anchor to the present moment on which the mind can rest and to which it can return. When you are conscious of your breath, you focus on the moment and there is no other place you can be.

How long will you stay present? That will depend on how long you are willing to stay awake.

So wake up to this moment and to this breath.

Before you move or think, embody the immediate meaning of yoga by uniting your mind and your body, the material and the intellectual, and take a deep breath in, relax and breathe out.

7.   UNVEIL

The moon's closeness to Earth has immediate effects on your life, ranging from oceanic tide fluctuations to the feminine cycle of life. You can think of Luna, the culprit of many fairy tale transformations, as your head, the dwelling place your mind. Your mind, with its jumping monkeys, soaring butterflies, and gushing river of thoughts, seems so tangible, yet so unattainable.

The sun, bright and present, which awakens you every morning, penetrates and reveals like the heart. Just as the heart pumps life into every region of the body, so the sun's presence is often overshadowed in its contribution to our psyche. Too far to reach and far too hot to touch, man admires and reveres the sun for its radiance, but it is admired from afar.

The influence is even more magnified with the coming of a solar eclipse, when the moon moves between the brightness of the sun and our planet Earth. For a moment your head will try and take over your heart. Often the mind is confused with a masculine quality of presence and stability, and the heart is identified as the feminine interaction of change. The rational scientific mind ignores insights from the heart. The mind, under the moon's influence, may articulate ideas, but their core begins much lower in the domain of the sun, the heart.

Feel deep into the center of your chest; notice the constant rhythm, or drumbeat, which sparked a vibration, igniting the synapses and allowing your brain to start producing thoughts. How often do your thoughts change? How quickly do you transition from one subject to another? Yet your heartbeat continues its movement, dancing to a rhythm that hardly wavers.

Solar eclipses are nature's way of bringing awareness to this phenomenon. As the sun comes through the shadow and your body reaches out to be touched by golden rays, you are offered a glimpse of your deep connection—a vision of the divine and a moment of utter joy. This is what the Tantric writings describe as the dance of consciousness and light, of sun and moon, and of heart and mind.

The moon is a pivotal part in the dance, just as thoughts are critical when we are to file our taxes. It's less about not thinking and more about enjoying the fullness of the thought (in other words, what does it feel like, what does it look like, how fast does it travel, and what shape is it). Recognizing its source is the ever-present consciousness in you that was there before you were born and after you die. So when you have a thought, feel it, touch it, and think nothing of it.

Let your sun shine. Let your heart rule. Your heart knows more than your head. Your heart takes its first beat before the mind awakens through blood flow and neuromuscular brain interaction. The heart has its own nervous center, and it processes emotions much faster than the head does. Situated deep within this four-chamber organ of blood circulation lies your inner light and true core. You are as bright as the sun, so run outside, and offer your heart in dance. Who knows what the eclipse will release from your mind?

Moment by moment, breath draws the mind and body, sun and moon, and yin and yang together as one. This breath crosses the bridge of separation between the mind and heart to find the central channel between the *ida* [the right nostril] and *pingala* [the left nostril].

Did you watch your breath in the last chapter? Do it now for five minutes and be a witness for your body.

Observe if the breath creates an eclipse around your heart, affecting how you sense the separateness of mind and heart. Don't just breathe. Breathe through to your core. Inhale deep down into the belly and relax. Let your belly become round as you fill the lower ribs with oxygen. Fill your body with this life energy; fill your moment with the play of light and consciousness.

In his *sutras*, Patanjali writes, "*svasa parsvasayor gati vicchedah pranayamah*" [when the movements of inhalation and exhalation are controlled, that is Pranayama]. Let the breath be gentle, relaxed, and even, without agitation. Let the breath move the body. Let your breath move your fingers as you turn the page.

8.   ENERGY

Within yogic teaching, breath is a mere reflection of *prana,* the Sanskrit work for the energy that keeps us alive and runs in the veins of all life. You can manipulate this life force for strength most deeply through *uddi-yana bandha* [flying upward lock]. This lock central point lies within the lower abdominal muscles, slightly below the navel. You use the abdominal muscles to draw the lower belly in and then pull the belly up, locking the belly and massaging the lower lobes of the heart. When your movements move from this center, you can access untapped physical possibilities, from complicated ballet movements to martial arts feats of strength.

As Sarah stands in the ring listening to Mona, the tall dark-haired horse trainer, and watching the beautiful steed in front of her, she considers the paradox of the moment. Since childhood, large animals, like the horse in the ring, have always frightened her, and she has never explored why.

"By facing our anxieties and internal fears, we are able to experience and relax despite the tension," Mona explains to Sarah. "Grounded in the principles of body awareness and breath, we stay in the moment, accept fear, accept anxiety, accept failure, and, thus, are no longer held back by them."

Sarah looks at Mona amazed. She never considered that an interaction with a horse would evoke proverbs from her own yoga teacher's classes. His words from the class filter through her mind.

"Face your fear; it will disappear."

"Be present in this moment. Allow all feelings to appear, and through breath, your body will show you what it needs."

As Sarah listens to the trainer and reflects on what she has learned, she finds the courage to face her fear.

"A horse is a very sensitive animal," Mona says with a smile while looking into Sarah's eyes. "Horses feel energy and respond to energy. By directing energy from your core body—from your belly button region to the top of your inner thighs—you will be able to control this eight-hundred-pound magical creature."

Sarah's face reacts to Mona's word, indicating a mixture of disbelief, surprise, and fear. The reaction causes Mona to smile even wider, exposing the dimples in her cheeks.

"It's very simple," Mona insists.

Mona turns to face the stallion. Within an instant, the horse begins to gallop around the outside wall of the ring. Though standing ten feet away, circling in place without any physical contact with the horse, Mona is in complete control of the stallion's movements.

"Notice how I am directing him with my belly," she instructs. "I don't have to use my hands or my stick. I am sending him a command through my body. If I want the horse to change direction, I draw my core toward its head."

Mona moves her body toward the stallion's face, and immediately the horse changes direction.

"If I want to make the horse go faster, I walk closer to him."

With obvious awareness, Mona steps closer to the enchanting animal, and he speeds up. As Sarah watches this unfold, her face beams with childlike disbelief. Mona returns to her guest's side and encourages her to try it.

"Relax your body, and feel your breath in your belly," she explains. "As you exhale, feel your lower belly contracting, and from that point in your body, direct your energy outward. You can exaggerate if you like, but it should feel as if your belly is sending a beam of light toward its tail."

Feeling self-conscious, but remembering that this concept was very similar to a position Sarah's yoga teacher had called uddiyana bandha, Sarah directs her navel at the horse, and within seconds, the horse moves around the ring.

"That's it," Mona cheers. "You're a natural. You should come and help me train them next time."

Our breath and our bodies communicate so much more than our words. The quality of our posture, the fullness of our breath offers a chance for our core truth to express itself. The tone of our voice, the decision we make, affect our lives and those around us. Stand firm and deliver, with all you can, from your core truth. Would you live any other way?

9. EXPRESS OR REPRESS?

What do you do when you are angry or fearful? Do you shut down and close yourself off from the world around you, immersed in your own thoughts of fury and despair? Or do you move to shed off the negative feeling by directing the energy outward, screaming at the sales clerk who happened to also be in a bad mood?

Often you deny yourself the full expression of your emotions. You can express positive emotions, but you repress the negative ones. The paradox is that emotions are like patterns of weather in the physical domain of life. Sometimes you have a clear, sunny day, and sometimes you have a dark-clouded moment. If you allow your emotions to move and interact as weather patterns, you could relax deeper into the moment and carry no residue of unexpressed tension.

This concept is exemplified in a story I tell my yoga students:

Two yoga students walk along the Himalayas back to their yoga shala [school]. Soon they arrive at the bank of the Ganges River. An older woman sitting by the water edge asks them if they could help her cross the wide river. Gladly, they place her on their shoulders and carry her to the other side, where she goes on her way and they continue on theirs.

A few hours later, one of the friends turns to the other and says, "We are neophytes, and we are not allowed any contact with women. Do you think we will face any problems back at the shala?"

The second student looks at his friend and replies, "We left the woman at the side of the river. Why are you still carrying her?"

When you try to assuage the emotional hurricane in the body as the first student is doing in the story above, you create mental impressions. As a modern example, say your boss and coworkers disparage a project you have worked on for weeks. As you take in the criticism, you can feel your belly tighten with shame, your heart harden for protection, and your mind race with excuses.

"My boss has no communication skills."

"My coworkers have no taste."

"I know I am good."

These thoughts are an attempt to grab personal assurance of your existence and worth. Your thinking creates your own sinking by perpetuating the veil you place on your true self and your sense of the cosmic connection between you and those who criticize you.

How can you express your frustration while maintaining this sense of connection? And what would it look like physically to listen to their comments fully while assessing what is true and what is not, and still shine as who you truly are?

Instead of tensing when the barrage of criticism comes, relax into your breath, rest your belly and your shoulders, and feel completely the size and shape of the sensations running through you. What is the texture of emotions? Is it rough and edgy, coarse and pricked? Feel your body fully, as if you are floating in a lake. You see the pollen-covered surface and gaze deeper into the darkening water, where light particles begin to fight their way through dense water molecules, gaze deep through your breathe, until you can see to the bottom of the lake.

Grounded through breath, you can focus on the others in front of you. When do they breathe? When do their bodies clench and close? When does their breath quicken or slow? Can you maintain eye contact without staring and making the other person feel self-conscious?

Yoga practice helps develop the inner tools to stay centered and directed, yet soft and pliable. Such a quality influences every environment you are in from your home setting to a crowded restaurant. With practice, you will find that your calm breath awareness is transferred to any environment you are in.

10. LET GO OF YOUR ANGER

Fear and anger follow one another, like lovers caught in a battle of betrayal. Your egocentric self, the mind, resists surrendering to the eternal self within, defying the encompassing energy that fuels the dance of your existence. The emotional toll of being afraid when faced with a new edge in a posture, a miscommunication in your relationship, or a challenging experience in your life triggers your sense of inadequacy by illuminating what you lack in skill or intellect and uncovers your habitual patterns of thinking and acting. In order to rid yourself of these negative thoughts, you either internalize your anger or extend it out to the universe, usually directing at the people around you or those who are close to your heart.

To illustrate this principle, I like to tell a story about a yoga student to my yoga class:

A young yoga student, who was traveling throughout India, spent time studying with many different teachers, searching for enlightenment.

One day, arriving at the home of a new teacher, the yoga student begins to explain what he has learned.

"The self, the mind, and all sentient beings—they really do not exist. The real truth behind phenomenon is emptiness. There is no attainment, no delusion, no gurus, and no mediocrity. There is nothing to give and nothing to take away."

After listening to this speech while smoking, the teacher suddenly hits the young man with his bamboo pipe.

The young boy becomes extremely angry and demands, "Why did you do that?"

"If nothing exists," replies the teacher, "then where is this anger coming from?"

Much like the young student in this story, a common worldview is to separate your own reality from the reality of the objects and events. From this perspective, you can avoid moments that challenge you or you can fight through them, pushing and struggling against the odds. It creates a tension that blocks your ability to expand your awareness and focus on being present in the moment.

In a class I attended, Geshe (title equally to a Doctorate of Divinty) Michael Roach, one of a select few who have spent twenty-five years studying deep in Tibet, and the first westerner to receive Geshe title, illustrates this dilemma by posing a question to his class:

"What am I holding in my hand?" he asks, raising his pen high into the air.

Feeling self-conscious at the obvious answer, the room wavers in confusion before someone says, "It's a pen."

"That's right," Rosh comments with a smile. "This is a pen."

The uncomfortable unease is broken by soft giggles.

"My partner and I recently added a new member to our home," he continues. "A beautiful, small pug puppy named Shree. As I was writing, Shree sniffed at it and began to chew on it with her young teeth. For me it was a pen, a writing tool, but for Shree, it was a toy, something to chew on and play with. So who is right? Is it a pen or is it a toy?"

If there was an awkward silence after the first question, the discomfort looms as they ponder the second.

"It's neither," an anonymous answerer feebly attempts from the depth of the crowd.

"It's still a pen," remarks a young man, dressed in flowing white robe.

"I am not sure how many will get what I am about to say," Rosh continues, beaming with childlike glee at the curious eyes seated before him. "My teacher suggests that one has to hear the explanation one thousand times before one gets it. We think of this pen as a pen for its own sake. However, the pen-ness of this object does not arise from its own nature. We assign the nature to this object, much as Shree assigns a different quality to the same object. It's this suggestion that the object is created for its own sake that causes confusion, ignorance, and suffering. This pen is not a pen for its own benefit. We assign the value to all things around us. When we can see how we make these choices, we will cease to hang on to the values and realize that all life rises from a deeper source, a source to which we are constantly connected."

The art of practicing breath juxtaposes your judgmental point-of-view of right and wrong with your experience of divinity, which can't be reduced to good or bad. As your breath awareness deepens, your jaw softens, your smile widens, and your outlook clears so that you see to what you are paying attention. By softening this *attention* and no longer placing the mind or the body *at tension*, you experience the choice of relaxation. When you stay present and open to *all* of the emotions, physical sensations, and thoughts that come up, and then choose to feel beyond them, you may experience your true self, or the causal body, which is of the same quality in everything. With your breath as an anchor, you experience the challenge of a lesson in letting go from which you can grow and expand your awareness. Yet as long as you choose to hold onto separate values and remain ignorant of your eternal connectedness, fear and anger will reside in your heart.

So let whatever holds you back go. Let it go, and trust in the process to move beyond it.

11. SHOCK

After yoga class, I walk out into a cool breeze. The shifting wind descends from the north, an early sign of summer's end, and cools my heated body. Evaporated sweat lifts off my skin, creating smoke spirals. I like to think of this smoke as tension melting off of my body.

The yoga class I came from had been inspirational, bringing me to the edge of my suffering and my desire to be in control. I had learned to dance with my breath, which flowed from the teacher's constant reminder to be aware of the fullness of our being.

"If you need to rest, rest," he said. "Do more when you can do more, but do less when you feel restless. Let go of your tension. Smile. Don't frown."

As I remember his words, I enter the city park, trying to recall the various idioms and metaphors he had painted.

"Your issues live in your tissues," his accented voice sings. "Let your body heat so they can bubble to the surface. Come here now. You know how your body wants to move—"

Suddenly, something knocks me to the ground.

Feeling shocked and confused, I try to turn my head and see what has caused me to stumble. A forceful knee presses itself into the center of my back, and a strong hand presses my nose into the soft grass. The taste of the dirt in my teeth and the horror of realizing I am being attacked send my body into shivers.

"Give me all your money," a voice demands.

"Take my bag," I say, remembering I left my wallet in my car. "That's all I have."

I can feel the shaking in my voice and the tears that are building in my eyes.

"It'll be OK," the voice in my head cautions. "It will be OK."

As I feel the bag being ripped from my shoulder, I surrender to my physical sensations. I want the hurt to go away, yet I also want to lash out and inflict pain. I want the taste in my mouth to sweeten, yet I want to scream out profanity and curse my attacker with a venom I never realized I possessed. In the midst of scanning my body, I realize that my anger is justified, but that feeling the anger has made me weak and made me shut down. Slowly I find my breath, which grounds me in this experience and allows me to channel my adrenaline.

"There is no money here," I tell him calmly.

I feel my attacker's knee press even deeper into my back. Through my own pain, I feel my attacker's beating heart. I concentrate more and notice that he is trying to disguise his voice and the words coming out of his mouth are shaking. I realize he is afraid.

Not being able to connect with his eyes or breath, I soften more.

"I know," I say to comfort him, "but it's OK. You're OK. Don't worry. We can go to my car. How much money do you need? We can try and arrange for you to get it."

Suddenly, I feel the pressure on my spine is gone, and I hear his footsteps as he runs away from the scene. In the silence of the night, the wind is the sole witness to the occurrence.

Smelling of grass and licking the earth from my teeth, I start to cry—for my own pain, for my attacker's sense of despair, for the people who are mugged and raped every day, and for the suffering that occurs in the world. I cry without any sadness for myself. I cry, and as tears flow down my face, my body begins to shiver and I hear myself begin to laugh.

I notice a glow around my body that extends far into the night. As much as I cry, I also laugh, and my body surrenders to fullness all around me, the same fullness that inspired Rumi's poems. As my emotions subside, I bring my palms together. I feel the interaction of two energies—mine and my attacker's. I offer up my fear, my panic, and my love. I bow my head, wipe my eyes, pick up my yoga bag, and walk back to my car.

12. BALANCING ACT

You are a Buddha. You are a being of knowledge.

This thought might cause you to say to yourself, "Well, I don't know quantum physics," "I don't know Sanskrit," or "I don't know how to put a car together." Quantum physics, Sanskrit, and mechanics are learned information, which appeals to your ego. Learning these concepts persuades your mind that you are becoming better, as though you are a separate entity and could be better than something else.

There is another kind of knowledge, which is not learned, but discovered, and not taught but explored. You can learn to read notes and where keys on the piano are to play those notes, but unless you touch, that is connect with, the keys, you will miss out of the music, and there is a beautiful song—the sounds of harmony—that can play through you.

A Buddha is someone who knows his or her deep, unique song that originates from the central musical source. A Buddha knows his or her deep purpose and inner light. Such knowledge isn't gained in a classroom or from a book; it can't be bought, sold, traded, or scanned. It is a knowledge that is always with you, but you are not always aware of it and in tune with it. You know, and yet you don't know, and when you discover and experience what it is that you didn't know, you will laugh at yourself.

For example, there is a word in Chinese—*mu*—that signifies "nothing" or "emptiness." It is an important component in Buddhist philosophy Truth is considered no-thing. Buddhist followers explore this concept using *koans*, or parables, like the following:

One day, a yoga master was asked, "Does a dog have a Buddha nature?"

The yoga master smiled and uttered, "Mu."

These koans urge you to forget what you know or don't know and move beyond the rational enclosed boundaries of the mind. You can restore the balance between the mind and the body, and your ego and your inner self. You can push yourself to a higher awareness.

As you grow in skill in yoga, these challenges will become balancing acts, where the mind and body struggle for control.

As the yoga class begins the balancing series, Daniel realizes it is going to be difficult and he wonders if he will be able to do it.

"It is easy to stand on two legs," says Dina, the instructor. "It builds courage to stand on one leg. Slowly, raise your right knee to your chest and either work with the knee or work with your big toe as you extend your leg."

Dina walks through the heated bodies, lending a hand to balance those who seem to need it the most.

"Falling is a learning process," she explains, "so relax, and if you fall, rise back."

Trying to keep his eyes focused on one point, Daniel's body shakes internally. He is trying hard to keep his balance on one leg. It is all a physical exercise for him at this point. His toes grasp against the mat, his face clenches in effort, and his breath titters from fast to erratic.

"Let your breath be soft, smooth, and flowing," Dina instructs.

Her voice swirls around Daniel's body as he attempts to follow her advice. His body reaches its breaking point, and he drops his leg. "I suck," the judging mind jumps into action. "Look at her, she is better than you."

"You might fall seven times," the instructor encourages, "but I promise you, you will get up on the eighth."

Daniel closes his eyes, relaxes his shoulders, and as his eyes regain focus, lifts his leg again.

"All you can do is try," he assures himself.

"Your body is only a temporary experience," Dina lectures while supporting a muscular male student. "As you balance, find the courage to go beyond the body. Slowly take your leg or knee to the side. Try to look past the opposite shoulder.

"In a balance pose, you have a chance to find your true voice, the voice deep inside that knows where you came from and where you will go.

"Are you listening, or are you resisting by trying so hard? Don't try hard. Try easy.

"Slowly come back to center, release your fingers and point your toe if you can. Straighten the leg if it is not already straight."

While holding his leg up, Daniel listens to his breath more and discovers a deep calm beyond his usual attention to the superficial thoughts. He presses his heel on the floor deeper into the mat and feels his inner thigh creating space into which the lifted hip can drop. He points his toes with confidence, not a fearful deathlike clench.

"We want to control all things in our lives, but we can never control everything," Dina continues. "Balance is a temporary illusion of control. Why not loose control? Why not surrender because you are courageous and allow the universe to support you? Don't be so serious. Give yourself permission to fall, to be out of balance, and to be out of control. When we can do that, we can meet our challenges with humor and with a soft smiling expression," Dina says as she smiles.

The room laughs with her. Many students fall out of balance.

"OK, lift your other leg up. Uthita Hasta Padangustasana. One …"

Are you living a controlled life? You might think you have to change everything in order to be content. Or maybe you are waiting for that glorious moment when you will have all of the money you want, the right relationship, and the perfect kids.

Look around. This moment is perfect as it is. This is heaven right here.

You are the manifestation of divinity.

As you balance your checkbook, your relationships, or your body on your arms or your legs, you can open your breath and body to express your truth. You can relax your habits of thinking, acting, and managing by constantly expressing the deep awareness of *your* life. This is another way of looking at practice, the discovery of the unique expression you have in moving, talking and breathing.

13. MAGIC

On a train ride from Delhi to Calcutta, an Englishman spots the poet Rumi standing by a window and throwing dust from a pouch out the window.

"What are you doing?" he asks Rumi.

"You see this pouch of mine," Rumi says. "This pouch has magical dust powders. With these magical dust powders, I am making sure no tigers attack our train."

The Englishman looks out the window at the beautiful terrain before him, but he doesn't see any tigers.

"But there are no tigers out here," he says.

"It's some powerful stuff I have here," Rumi replies with a smile.

Like Rumi's pouch, there is magical stuff inside of you. I see it every day in my classes.

"I can't stand on my head," Laura tells me decisively outside the yoga studio.

Her body and the tone of her voice stand as firm as a Roman pillar while her eyes have a trickle of childish longing.

A warm, late-summer breeze moves between us, as if pushing us into experimentation.

"I don't know what it is. When I try it in the middle of the room, I am sure I am going to fall," she says, softening her position as she speaks. "I have tried it with a wall, and I will do it if there is a wall."

"See," I encourage. "You can stand on your head. Never say never."

"It's not the same, you know," she fires back. "A part of me wants to do the pose right there on my mat, but then I freeze, or I simply stop."

Laura carries herself well. Her five-foot frame beams an inner confidence that brightens up a room.

"That's natural," I explain, remembering when I first had learned the posture and for months I would come home and use the wall. "It's a practice, not a goal, so long as you try. You'll surprise yourself one day."

"One day?" Laura questions with a broad smile stretched across her face. "Do you know how old I am?"

"Age is of no matter. The late teacher Krishnamacharya was standing on his head every morning at the age of ninety-one."

"I'm sixty-eight years old." She responds unimpressed.

"Rather than provide years, we should provide days." I explain. "Imagine if I told someone I was 12,775 days old, which sounds much more impressive than thirty-five years. Yet, nothing prevents you from standing on your head."

"I am not sure I can handle all the weight on my forearms. I had an injury when I was younger, and I could not use the right arm for a few weeks. I don't want to hurt it again."

"I have seen you go into *bakasana* [a strong arm balance known as the crane pose] without any problems."

Smirking, Laura considers that thought for a moment.

"Why don't we work together and work up to the posture?" I suggest. "We can thus shift the mental block and help you gain more confidence to explore the pose on your own, when you choose, and anywhere in the room your heart desires."

We agree to meet the following morning.

"I'm warning you," she says as she walks toward her car, "I'm feeling a little anxious about it."

I offer her my smile and a simple namaste gesture. In my heart, I know that whether or not she stands on her head, she'll have a different attitude about the subject when she emerges from savasana.

In most cases like Laura's, your fears are rooted in a misconception of your bodies or grounded in a negative experience you have had. Why is it that one negative consequence leaves a mark for years, while positive feedback has to be reassessed before it is internalized? Instead of limiting yourself when you fail, you should simply try again.

As the old Buddhist koan says, "We don't fail. We simply find ten thousand ways how *not* to do it."

14. INTENTION

A shift in consciousness has to occur before a shift in the body can happen. If you only change your physical body without delving into the depth of your emotions and thoughts, then you are going to face the same dilemmas again. If you only change what you do, you only change your behaviors and don't discover the full potential lying dormant inside you.

When you focus solely on the body, trying to mold it and change it to fit your desired image, you confine yourself to an end. Although setting goals is a needed element in growth and development, often you get boxed into your goals, or you set goals that far outweigh your capacity, thus you set yourself up for failure, disappointment, and ultimately, internal suffering.

Set your goals, and plan ahead, but come back to the moment by identifying your intention. Goals are the destination, like an island adventure, but the intention is how you approach these moments, like the wind that blows your sails. Sometimes the wind is gliding you along calm waters, sometimes it is rough and you feel you are about to tip over, and sometimes there is no wind at all. Do you jump for joy when the wind gusts softly, only to curse in fear and anger when it threatens to knock you over? Do you fall into despair when it disappears and you feel stuck?

Intentions help monitor moment-by-moment exchanges to keep our mind and body pure. How is your breath moving? Are you sitting straight, or are your shoulders drooping and is your chest closed? These are the exchanges of our inner world and the subtle body, and our outer world and the gross body. These exchanges offer valuable information that draws you outside of your limited point of view to recognize the fullness of every moment and thus uncover your true essence, which is the fullness of life.

In a far away forest lives a turtle that understands human speech. One afternoon he overhears a pair of hunters discussing their plans to return the next day and hunt turtles. Startled, the turtle begins to ponder solutions to his predicament. Slowly he devises a plan. He decides he will ask his two eagle friends to carry a branch in their talons that he will bite and they can carry him to the nearby forest.

After presenting the idea to his eagle friends, they agree. The eagles grab a hold of the branch, the turtle bites it, and off into the sky, they go.

As they fly over, the forest animals below begin to exclaim, "Look. A turtle is flying in the sky."

Choose your goals and actions mindfully. Fully aware that what you say has as much consequence as what you do. How would you choose your words and actions so that they might shine true, avoiding a fall from the sky?

Yet you get caught up in your goal setting, which is thinking rather than acting and demanding rather than appreciating. In the rush to reach your goals, you stiffen your body, shorten your breath, and react rather than respond to the challenges or joys that come your way. Rather than forgoing of your goals, can you explore the reasons behind them and navigate through the many options that are available to you? On the path, things can change, and at times you might discover a deeper good your actions can make, thus reforming your final goal. If you fail to appreciate the immediate moment and how it unfolds on the journey to reach the goal, you set yourself up to battle with your judgment.

For example, are you doing the pose correctly? If you care about the final goal of looking like a poster child for yoga, you tend to fight with your body and miss out on the process of feeling how bones move, how ligaments stretch, how the breath deepens, and how the mind centers and becomes clear. You may or may not get the leg behind the head, but your sense of self will enlarge to encompass someone else. You let go of the habitual ways of thinking and become more compassionate of your own experience, propelling you to be compassionate toward those who are unhappy, to disregard those who are wicked, to make friends with those who are truly happy, and to bask in the luminous light of those who are virtuous.

15. LIGHT YOUR FLAME

A yoga student asks his master, "What is enlightenment?"

"Eat when you are hungry; sleep when you are tired," she answers with a smile.

"But how do we reach enlightenment?"

"You want to reach enlightenment?" she replies. "To reach enlightenment all you need is to lighten up."

Think of the most exciting thing for which you have planned or trained. Feel in your body the thrill of putting those plans together or practicing for those hours. Savor the ardor with which you did them. Is it rich and creamy as warm chocolate fudge, is it fluffy and sweet as whipped cream, or is it as juicy and sticky as a melon? Taste that moment with all of your senses.

Remember the morning of the event, the morning of the trip, of the game, of the show, of the meeting. Recall the enthusiasm you felt in your body. Feel your heart racing as if were fueled with adrenaline. Notice the undivided attention in your eyes and the direction in your stride and speech. That day, your nervous system was a brightly shining fire of intention and enthusiasm.

The word *enthusiasm* finds its roots in the Greek words *en theos* which literally means "to have divine." When we prepare and involve ourselves fully in our actions, others feel the divine in us.

Patanjali refers to this quality in his second book, *Sadhana Pada [Book on Practice]*. Sutra 43 *"kayendriya-siddhir asuddhi-ksayat tapasah"* can be translated, "Through enthusiasm, we destroy the impurities of mind and body." In other words, let your enthusiasm clear away the doubt, and let the light of inspiration fuel your activity.

Patanjali urges you to bring this attitude to every moment in your life, not just the special ones. What might happen if you brought enthusiasm to brushing your teeth, to washing the dishes, to speaking with your children, to interacting with strangers, or to your daily practice?

To live your life fully in each moment is to bring enthusiasm into the smallest things you encounter and experience. In such a way, you can share your divinity and tap into the source of happiness.

16. TRANSFORMATION

In a small studio, a varied group of practitioners sits absorbed in Nada-Yoga, the yoga of chanting. As the voices mingle together, the room fills with a sense of unity. At the end of the chant, Russ, the round-bodied chant leader, begins a story.

"Two brothers inherit ten million each and go out to different sections of the world. Twenty years later, they meet at a river's edge.

"'You want to see what I have been doing for the last twenty years?' asks one of the brothers.

"'Of course,' replies the latter.

"The first brother closes his eyes to meditate and suddenly levitates himself off of the ground. Maintaining his meditation, he floats across the river to the other side, where he slowly lowers down, opens his eyes, and smiles.

"His brother crosses over the bridge, walks to his brother, slaps him across the face, and says, 'This is all you have done for the last twenty years?'"

Scattered giggles and a few hearty laughs resound in the studio. Russ transitions from the story to the heart of its message.

"So you have a beautiful voice," he says, preaching with his deep baritone voice. "You have a beautiful body. You make lots of money. Now what? How does it serve the people around you and the world around you? How will you take your practice and offer it to the universe? How will your practice change when you incorporate that principle into your activity? How will your interactions, your business relations, and your family ties expand when you become mindful of this? Think of that as we chant 'Om Namah Shiva' [I bow to Shiva]. Let your voice be one with all voices."

The harmonium begins to pour out its sound, and Russ's voice twirls into an ascending variation of "Om Namah Shiva." As the class begins to follow the rhythm, the voices join in harmony. I notice how I am self-conscious about trying to make my voice sound as good as the other tones my ears hear.

"So what if I can't levitate over water," I remind myself.

The thoughts continue as I loose myself in the chant, and I realize how my thoughts compare me to the others and make me feel separate from them. Ironically as the chant continues, it validates that separate sense identity. As our voices commingle and become one sound of various flavors, I feel a distinctive glow.

I open my eyes in surprise to notice how clearly I can see some of the faces in the room.

"What was it that Rumi wrote?" I ask myself. "'Rather than be with everyone, become everyone. When you are that many, you are no-thing, you are empty.'"

In chanting, sharing one's voice with the universe, I catch a glimpse of such a connection. It is a moment perfectly present in breath when the mind and body relax into sound.

We are all here, chanting together, twirling with sound like a dervish twirling in dance, and loosing ourselves to find ourselves.

17. TOUCH YOUR TOES

> Everything in the universe is only a weird dance of electrified nothingness.
>
> —Tom Robbins, American author

Take off your shoes and dance. Take off your socks and wiggle your toes. Allow winds of invisible currents to flow through your feet and up your entire body.

Your feet carry you wherever you go, and much like your breath, they are taken for granted. Stretching and exploring the wide range of motion the muscles of your feet provide a new sensory realm for the body, as well as a healing quality to the soul. How far can you spread your toes apart? Can you consciously control your feet, or are they a territory you wish to avoid, to ignore, and to escape?

If breath connects, then feet ground. Every nerve ending in the body ends here. For centuries travelers have been searching across continents and oceans for a map guide to health, and the feet are the key. With Eastern healing modalities gaining wide acceptance in the West, you may have read about, or given or received some form of a foot massage, recognizing not only the physical calmness it provides, but also the internal digestive aid and mental invigoration such interaction can exert on your overall being.

Yogis and yoginis have focused on using the feet as a source of good health for centuries. For example, students of yoga "fist" their toes to ease daily tension and "dance," breathing and moving, as a way of uniting themselves with the world around them.

Dance is a practice that flows with physical movements, social caring, vocal melodies, and/or intellectual ponderings. Through it, you can connect with the mind and body, the masculine and feminine, the sun and moon, and yin and yang.

Practiced throughout India by children and aging adults, *Surya Namaskar* [Sun Salutation], which is a sequence of postures coordinated with breath, is the oldest form of spiritual exercise after spontaneous dancing. Sun

Salutation activates the proprioceptor neural facilitator [PNF], which returns the body to a parasympathetic, or relaxed, nervous state. This simple practice balances blood flow, initiates movements in all of the major muscle groups, and instigates a full range of motion in the major joints of the body.

To practice Sun Salutation, stand up tall with your feet together and arms by your side. Inhale, and lift your arms over your head. Truly take in the depth of this moment. Exhale, and release your body to the foundation beneath you and put your hands on the floor by your feet. Inhale, and step back with your left leg. Keep this beautiful breath in your body, and step back into, *urdhava dandasana* [high push-up pose], slowly bend your elbows as you exhale into *chataranga dandasana* [low push-up pose]. Inhale lower your belly to the floor and lift your chest into *bhujangasana* [cobra pose]. Smile. Exhale, and push off, get strong and get long, and move into *adho mukha svanasana* [downward-facing dog pose]. Inhale, and bring your left foot between your hands. Exhale, and step its partner as you move deeper into *uttanasana* [standing forward bend]. Inhale, and raise arms over head, greet your day with glee. Exhale, arms come down as you settle back into your moment, only to repeat the process again leading with the right leg. Repeat sequence again and again, as many as you like, as many as 108, and as little as 1. Let your body tell your mind when to stop. The more you relax into your breath, the more you will find yourself completing.

At that moment you are breathing with the entire universe.

EPILOGUE

You don't have to get on a rubber mat to do yoga.

You don't need to wear any special clothing or do any pretzel postures.

You can allow your perceptions to soften right now and become conscious of your breath.

It is the same air that every other human being takes in. It is the same oxygen that plants process, animals partake in, and the ocean mingles with.

Your breath is your connection, to connect is to unite, and to unite is yoga. You can connect with your family, your friends, the trees, the animals, or yourself. You can do it right now as you connect with your breath.

Remember to laugh about it. Every time you loose the thread come back to your breath, the thread will appear instantly.

Two cows are standing in a field.

One cow turns to the other and says, "Are you afraid of mad cow disease?"

"No," says the second cow. "I'm a squirrel."

53

Don't confuse who you are. You are more than your name on your driver's license and more than the title behind or in front of your name on that driver's license.

You are unique, because there will never be another person like you. You are special, because you have your own gifts and talents to share in this life. You are not unique and special because you are better, but rather because you exist, and the same is true of the person next to you.

Let your practice help you discover your unique expression of the connection we all share.

Let your song play true and loud.

Namaste.

978-0-595-42595-2
0-595-42595-X

www.ingramcontent.com/pod-product-compliance
Lightning Source LLC
Chambersburg PA
CBHW020404290526
45785CB00005B/2433